School Based & Pediatric Occupational Therapy Resource Series:

Groups to Facilitate Motor , Sensory and Language Skills 2

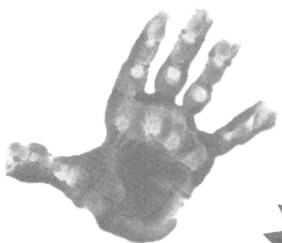

New! Updated Version with Sensory Integration and OT Practice Domain Framework.

By: S. Kelley, OTD, OTR/L

Purple Toes Books

School Based & Pediatric Occupational Therapy Resource Series:
Groups to Facilitate Motor, Sensory and Language Skills 2

S. Kelley

By S Kelley, OTD OTR/L
First Edition
© Purple Toes Books
Http:\\www.purpletoesbooks.com
U.S.A

Dedication

This book is gratefully and gracefully dedicated to all the families and team members that I have shared in my journey.

This is for you.

Acknowledgements

This book and my work as an occupational therapist are made possible by the support and love of many wonderful people. I would like to thank my mentors, colleagues, and team members over the years, over the miles. Each experience has been unique and rewarding and I am thankful to have shared them with you.

I would like to acknowledge my husband for his unwavering support and love. To my parents and grandparents, you have provided me with the foundation for which I have remained grounded.

Special Thanks

To my son. Without your life, love and perseverance I would never know my own strength.

Let Go. Let God.

About the Author

Dr. S. Kelley, OTD, OTR/L currently practices as a pediatric occupational therapist in the school setting. She has facilitated the participation and skill growth for students in both regular education and special education programs. With a background as both an early childhood teacher and occupational therapist, Dr. Kelley has a unique and specialized perspective of education for students. Dr. Kelley specializes in the treatment of students in the early childhood self contained special education classes. After nearly 15 years of practice, Dr. Kelley decided to create resources for the school based and pediatric therapist to help facilitate effective and efficient practice. These resources reflect both the OT Practice Framework (AOTA, 2008) and the Common Core Curriculum (Common Core Standards Initiative, 2012). These resources were then made available in alternative formats for families and parents as a response from families and co-workers.

Dr. Kelley holds a Bachelor of Arts in Early Childhood Education from Clemson University and a Bachelor of Science in Occupational Therapy from University of Wisconsin-Milwaukee. She also holds a Professional Master's and Doctorate degree in Occupational Therapy from Boston University. Dr. Kelley is registered nationally as a specialist in pediatric occupational therapy.

About the *Resource Series* from Purple Toes Books

The purpose of the *Resource Series*, in various formats, is to provide the reader a collection of practice, easy-to-use activities to assist with various motor, language and social skills. The *Resource Series* is a result of over 15 years of practice in pediatric occupational therapy. Over the course of my practice, I have created, developed, borrowed, collaborated, brainstormed, altered and modified countless activities and tasks. I decided to create a written series of my favorite activities as I use them, in the classroom, in the home or in the clinic.

Although I encourage you to read this book and independently apply the activities and/or interventions in your daily practice, classroom or life, please remind yourself that professionals are available to help you if you need advice or direction. These books are designed to be easy-to-use, but various professionals can help with modifications or adaptations if you need them.

Table of Contents

Occupational Therapy in School Setting

Definition of OT in the School Environment

Occupational therapists promote functional activities and engagement of daily routines. Areas of occupation including, but are not limited to: work, play, leisure, social participation, ADL, IADLs and Education. According to IDEA, occupational therapy services in the school setting are a support services for students identified eligible for special education services. Under Part B of IDEA (2004), services are provided through the individual education plan (IEP) to promote academic success and social participation , to access, progress and participation in the educational environment in the least restrictive environment (AOTA, 2012). Under IDEA's Part B (2004) Regulation the Definition of Occupational Therapy includes the following components:

1. Services must be provided by a qualified occupational therapist
2. Services may "improve, develop or restore functions impaired or lost through illness, injury or deprivation"
3. Services may "improve the ability to perform tasks for independent functioning if functions are impaired or lost"
4. Services may "prevent, through early intervention, initial or further impairment or loss of function" (IDEA, 2004)

OT Goals & Outcomes

Through direct, collaborative and consultative services, occupational therapist create individualized goals with focus on outcomes related to:

1. General Classroom Skills/Accessibility/Participation
2. Playground and Sports Accessibility/Participation
3. School Based Self Help Skills
4. Social Participation in the School Setting
5. Mobility in the educational environment
6. Social Emotional Learning
7. Assistive technology in the educational setting

8. Sensory Regulation
9. Pre-vocational and Vocational Needs in the educational setting

Specific Services Occupational Therapists in the School Setting

- Evaluate students' strengths and weaknesses
- Identify modifications to promote participation
- Provide direct interventions to facilitate function and skill acquisition
- Collaborate and consult with teachers and staff regarding student needs to access his/her educational environment

All Student Support Systems

Occupational therapists in the school setting may provide support services for students with and without disability. This is done through early intervening services, including Response to Intervention.

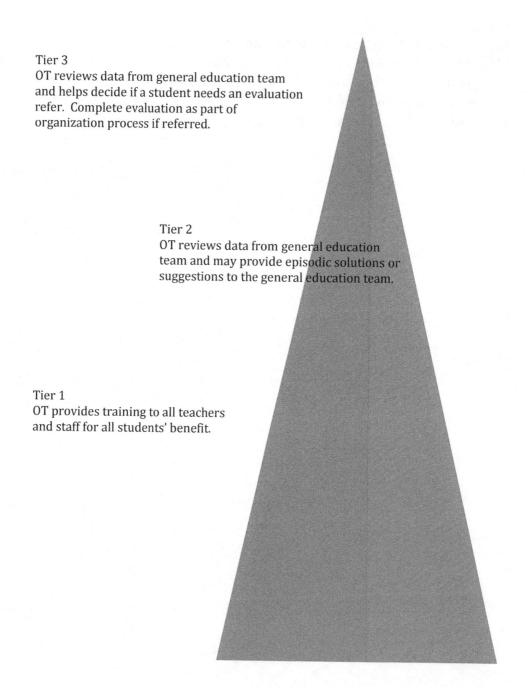

Tier 3
OT reviews data from general education team and helps decide if a student needs an evaluation refer. Complete evaluation as part of organization process if referred.

Tier 2
OT reviews data from general education team and may provide episodic solutions or suggestions to the general education team.

Tier 1
OT provides training to all teachers and staff for all students' benefit.

Resources' Reflection of the OT Practice Framework: Domain and Process

(AOTA, 2008).

This book provides a group method to provide services for students with and without disability. Below are the components reflected in the OT Practice Framework (AOTA, 2008) that are potential outcomes of the group treatment.

After the students' occupational profile has been developed, this group serves as the intervention plan, implementation and review within the intervention process. The intervention process includes the following (AOTA, 2008):

- Plan: Guides the actions of the OT and is based on the students' priorities
- Interventions: Carried out actions that address performance skills, patterns, context, activity demands and client factors that are impacting performance
- Review: Allow for revisions in the plan and actions

It should be noted, all interventions have the primary goal to achieving the primary outcome of engagement in occupation to support participation. (AOTA, 2008)

Areas of Occupation
Education
Play
Leisure
Social Participation

Performance Skills
Motor Skills
     Posture (Stabilizes, Aligns, Positions)
     Mobility (Walks, Reaches, Bends)
     Coordination (Coordinates, Manipulates, Flows)
     Strength & Effort (Moves, Transport, Lifts, Calibrates, Grips)
     Energy (Endures, Paces)
Process Skills

Energy (Paces, Attends)
Knowledge (Chooses, Uses, Handles, Heeds, Inquires)
Temporal Organization (Initiates, Continues, Sequences, Terminates)
Organizing Space & Objects (Searches, Gathers)

Intervention Plan for Groups

Occupational Therapy Intervention Approach
Create/Promote – performance skills, activity demands
Establish/Restore – performance skills
Maintain – performance skills, activity demands

Mechanism for Service Delivery
OT will provide the intervention with the support of additional team members which may include a speech language pathologist, physical therapist, teacher and/or support staff in the classroom

Each group should be delivered one time; however, the teacher or team may decide to expand the concept if additional practice is warranted. Additionally, group plans are designed to be delivered weekly. Groups should be implemented for about twenty to thirty minutes.

Outcome Measures & Types of Outcomes

Long term goal is to promote and facilitate the engagement in occupation. "Engagement in occupation (education or play) to support participation is the broad outcome of intervention that is designed to foster performance in desired and needed occupations or activities" (AOTA, 2008, p. 627).

Each group focus on the outcome of occupational performance (access to education).

Therapeutic Use of Self
The therapist uses his/her own personality, insight, perception and judgments throughout the intervention. Each group requires the therapist to use his/herself to be a part of the intervention.

Therapeutic Use of Occupations and Activities
Each group uses the following -

Occupational-Based Activity: Use of actual occupations as part of the intervention to support the outcome

Purposeful Activity: Use of goal-directed behaviors and activities in a therapeutically designed task

Resources' Connection to the Common Core Curriculum
(National Governors Association Center for Best Practices & Council of Chief State School Officers, 2010).

It is the goal of this group treatment to support the Common Core Curriculum. Below are components connected to the Common Core Curriculum. Due to the nature of the Common Core Domain, only broad standards in Kindergarten are provided. Please see the Common Core Curriculum for additional grades.

English Language Arts

ENGLISH LANGUAGE ARTS STANDARDS: LANGUAGE

CCSS.ELA.Literacy.L.K.1a	Print many upper and lower case letters.
CCSS.ELA.Literacy.L.K.1b	Use frequently occurring nouns and verbs
CCSS.ELA.Literacy.L.K.1c	Form regular plural nouns orally by adding /s/ or /es/
CCSS.ELA.Literacy.L.K.1d	Understand and use question words
CCSS.ELA.Literacy.L.K.1e	Use frequently occurring prepositions
CCSS.ELA.Literacy.L.K.1f	Produce and expand complete sentences in shared language
CCSS.ELA.Literacy.L.K.4a	Identify new meanings to new or familiar words
CCSS.ELA.Literacy.L.K.5a	Sort Common objects into categories
CCSS.ELA.Literacy.L.K.6	Use words and phrases acquired through conversations, reading and being read to

ENGLISH LANGUAGE ARTS STANDARDS:SPEAKING AND LISTENING

CCSS.ELA-Literacy.SL.K.1	Participate in collaborative conversations with diverse partners about topics with peers and adults
CCSS.ELA-Literacy.SL.K.1a	Follow rules for discussion (listen to others, taking turns)
CCSS.ELA-Literacy.SL.K.1b	Continue conversation through multiple exchanges
CCSS.ELA-Literacy.SL.K.2	Confirm understanding of text read aloud or information presented orally or through other media by asking and answering questions

CCSS.ELA-Literacy.SL.K.3	Ask and answer questions in order to seek help, get information, or clarify something misunderstood
CCSS.ELA-Literacy.SL.K.4	Describe familiar people, places, things and events with assistance
CCSS.ELA-Literacy.SL.K.5	Add drawings or visuals to provide additional information/details
CCSS.ELA-Literacy.SL.K.6	Speak audibly and express thoughts, feelings, and ideas

ENGLISH LANGUAGE ARTS STANDARDS:READING:FOUNDATIONAL SKILLS

CCSS.ELA.Literacy.RF.K.1a	Follow words from left to right, top to bottom, page to page
CCSS.ELA.Literacy.RF.K.1b	Recognize that spoken words are represented in written form

ENGLISH LANGUAGE ARTS STANDARDS: WRITING

CCSS.ELA.Literacy.W.K.1	Use a combination of drawing, dictating and writing to compose an opinion about the name of a book and preference about it
CCSS.ELA.Literacy.W.K.2	Use a combination of drawing, dictating and writing to create details about a topic
CCSS.ELA.Literacy.W.K.3	Use a combination of drawing, dictating and writing to narrate a single event about a topic
CCSS.ELA.Literacy.W.K.5	With assistance, respond to questions and suggestions to add details and strength writing
CCSS.ELA.Literacy.W.K.6	With assistance, explore a variety of digital tools to produce writing
CCSS.ELA.Literacy.W.K.7	Participate in shared research and writing projects
CCSS.ELA.Literacy.W.K.8	With assistance, recall information from experiences and gather information from sources to answer a question

Mathematics

MATHEMATICS:MEASUREMENT & DATA

CCSS.Math.Content.K.MD.A.1	Describe measurable attributes of objects
CCSS.Math.Content.K.MD.A.2	Directly compare two objects with measurable attributes
CCSS.Math.Content.K.MD.B.3	Classify objects in categories, count, and sort

MATHEMATICS:GEOMETRY

CCSS.Math.Content.K.G.A.1	Describe objects in the environment using names of shapes and use relative positions of these objects (spatial)
CCSS.Math.Content.K.G.A.2	Correctly name shapes
CCSS.Math.Content.K.G.A.3	Identify shapes

MATHEMATICS: COUNTING & CARDINALITY

CCSS.Math.Content.K.CC.A.1	Count to 100 by ones and tens
CCSS.Math.Content.K.CC.B.4	Understand the relationship between numbers and quantities.

Resources' & Sensory Integration Framework

Sensory Integration is defined as the organization of sensory input from one's environment and the responses one's body has as a result. It is a complex system that requires the nervous system to work in harmony together to interact with the environment and experiences within it.

Vestibular Response: Sensation from body regarding gravity and movement (knowing where one's head is in space)

Proprioception Response: Sensation from the body, muscles and joints (where the body "feels" itself in space

Tactile/Touch: Feeling through the body, hands, skin

Visual Sense: Seeing what's in space and distinguishing between various visual input

Auditory Sense: Hearing sounds in space and distinguishing between various sound input

Olfactory Sense: Smelling scents in space and distinguishing between various smells

Gustatory Sense: Tasting food in the mouth and distinguishing between different tastes (sour, sweet, etc)

Dysfunctional Response: Negative action or emotional response, lack of response or mismatched response

Adaptations and Modifications to Support Group Participation

Adaptation Defined
An adaptation is HOW the student accesses information in the classroom

Modification Defined
An modification is WHAT the student is expected to learn in the classroom.

Hierarchy of Accommodations & Modifications
Most special education students may need Level 2 & 3

Level	Accommodations	Modifications
1	All students complete same activities	No changes made to success criteria
2	All students complete same activities, additional support and reinforcement needed	No changes made to success criteria
3	All students complete basic concept, but significant changes made to how it is learned	Success criteria changed slightly
4	Students complete a smaller part of the expected activity	Success criteria based on individual needs
5	Students complete alternative activity	Success criteria based on individual needs

Adaptations for Group Sessions

Environment
- Provide organized and predictable space.
- Provide and reinforce rules and expectations.
- Create visual cues for rules and expectations.
- Create visuals for objects in the classroom.
- Remove visual clutter from space.
- Provide consistent expectations.
- Place students in a learning space that is removed from major distractions (doorway, pencil sharpener, distracting peers)
- Use visual behavior cue cards to redirect behaviors (stop, listen, look, quiet mouth)
- Distribute and encourage sensory tools for sensory seeking behaviors while seated
- Allow the use of noise cancelling headphones or earplugs for disruptions

Instruction
- Introduce basic concepts immediately before starting activity
- Reinforce concepts with frequent direction, redirection and questions
- Use manipulatives and movements
- Rephrase and repeat key concepts
- Reinforce vocabulary and concepts frequently
- Infuse discussion and instruction with desired concepts and vocabulary
- Reduce tasks to main concepts and components
- Focus on main concepts – eliminate extra information
- Move to a closer proximity to students when instructing

Fine Motor Specific

Experiment with:

Various grippers to improve control or grasping pattern
Weighted pencils for shaky marks (decreased motor control)
Vary the length or thickness of utensil
Vary type of utensil
Texture under paper (sandpaper)
Vary line sizes – start wider and get smaller
Raised line paper to cue base and top lines
Created raised line paper with glue
Skip every other line on paper
Enlarging paper to make fill in blanks larger
Experiment with adapted scissors – loop, mounted
Highlight desired fill in area
Provide stickers for a quick way to label work (instead of writing it)
Reduce written work required
Allow additional time to write
Provide near point from which to copy versus far point
Chair with side supports
Slant board
Label marker for spelling requirements
Recorder for oral responses vs written requirements
Word processor
Computer with voice recognition

Specific Motor, Sensory, & Language Skills Addressed During Interventions

Motor Skills

Bi-Lateral Integration – Use of two hands together
In Hand Manipulation Skills
Finger Isolation
Grasping Patterns
Midline Crossing
Trunk Elongation, Strength and Stability
Postural Control
Wrist Rotation, Strength and Control
Hand Dominance
Breath Support
Jaw Stabilization
Lip Closure
Tongue Elevation and Movements

Sensory Skills

Vestibular Input
Proprioceptive
Tactile
Visual
Auditory
Gustatory

Language Skills

Sound Recognition
Greeting Peers
Requesting Materials
Turn Taking

Introduction

Education and therapy goals are addressed in the classroom or clinic in a variety of ways: direct instruction, applied practice, independent performance and group experiences.   This book provides a group format to provide direct instruction and practice with underlying motor, sensory and language skills needed for classroom/clinic performance and participation. Benefits of the group experiences include:

1. Activities combine various domains needed for educational performance and participation. Domains addressed include occupational therapy, speech therapy, social work, physical therapy and educational. All fuse together to create fun opportunities for students to explore actions and body movements.

2. This group provides a model of educational based group models. Often it can be difficult to navigate and separate the educationally relevant versus clinically relevant. These activities are educationally based, developmentally sound and provide opportunity for play and experiences that are classroom and school based.

3. Groups are provided in the classroom with the direct support of classroom staff. It is encouraged that all team members be a part of the groups and that they expands and explore the concepts introduced when the therapist is no longer there.

Use of Puppetry

This program can be used with a puppet to provide a fun way to make greeting exchanges, improve eye contact and facilitate transitional changes. If you choose to use a puppet, designate a specific puppet in your classroom that correlates with groups done with this program. Name the puppet and allow him/her to be the mascot of the groups.

To use the puppet in this program, simply switch our the directions provided to include exchanges between the puppet and student versus the therapist and student.

Quick Reference for Needed Materials

Week 1

Materials:
Puppet (if using)
Individual Photos of students and staff in the classroom
Adapted choice boards of individual photos, if needed

Week 2

Materials:
Puppet (if using)
Playground ball or medium sized ball

Week 3

Materials:
Tissues
Ping Pong Balls

Week 4

Materials:
Bubbles
Cotton Balls
Straw

Week 5

Materials:
None

Week 6

Materials:
Scooterboard
Hula Hoop

Week 7

Materials:
Broomstick

Pinwheels

Materials:
Cube Chair

Materials:
Wind up toys
Baby jar with lids/or various jar with lids
M&M or desirable candy of choice

Materials:
Slinky
Rain Sticks

Materials:
Cups with pictures of choice under them (with matches not under cup)
Pair of pictures of choice
(Pictures may be related to theme)

Materials:
Circle shaped cereal
Pipe Cleaner
Yarn

Materials:
Puppet
Dry Noodles

Week 14

Materials:
Clothespins
Coffee Can
Tweezers
Strawberry Huller
Small pom pom/cotton

Week 15

Materials:
Theraputty
Pennies
Hairbeads
Coffee Can with a slit made for pennies

Week 16

Materials:
Shaving Cream
Towels
Plastic baby doll

Week 17

Materials:
Two buckets
6 sponges
Water in one bucket

Week 18

Materials:
Parachute
Stuffed Animal

Week 19

Materials:
Tug of War Rope

Week 20

Materials:
Bag of oranges cut into halves
Bowl
Paper Cups

Week 21

Materials:
Container with beans or sand
Small items (cars, plastic figures, etc. that are of child's interest)

Week 22

Materials:
Pillowcase
Beanbags
Obstacle Course

Week 23

Materials:
Green and red construction paper

Week 24

Materials:
Tactile ball (koosh, sensory, hacky sack)

Week 25

Materials:
Six beanbags
Bucket

Group Plans

Week 1

Focus:
Name Recognition
Greetings

Materials:
Puppet (if using)
Individual Photos of students and staff in the classroom
Adapted choice boards of individual photos, if needed

Method:
This is an introductory lesson designed to introduce the greeting process and expectations. The greeting process should be done every lesson to practice appropriate greetings and eye contact. If using a designated puppet, have the student greet the puppet. If not using a puppet, have the student greet the teacher or therapist.

Greeting

Sit in front of the students and greet each child individually. Provide augmentative communication or choice board for students that need assistance responding. Encourage eye contact as appropriate. Fleeting eye contact is acceptable is the intent is to provide joint attention.

Direct Instruction Example
Teacher/Therapist: "It's time for us to have group time. Hi Mrs. X!"
Teacher/Therapist: "Hi Mrs. X!" (or Hi puppet name)

Verbal Response
Teacher/Therapist: "It's time for us to have group time. Hi student x!"
Student X: "Hi Mrs. X. (or Hi puppet name)

Non Verbal Response
Teacher/Therapist: "It's time for us to have group time. Hi student x!"
Student X: Initiate eye contact, wave, smile in direction of teacher/therapist/puppet

Use of Communication Device
Teacher/Therapist: "It's time for us to have group time. Hi student x!"
Student X: Touch "Hi Mrs. X" on given choice board, communication device, Ipad, etc

Activity: Self Recognition

After all students have been greeted and have provided a response, continue to the expanded activity.
Show the students a picture of a peer.

Direct Instruction Example
Teacher/Therapist: "Who is this?"
Teacher/Therapist: "It's Me."
Teacher/Therapist: "What's your name"
Teacher/Therapist: "My name is x" "I am X". etc

Verbal Response
Teacher/Therapist: "Who is this?"
Student in Picture: "It's Me."
Teacher/Therapist: "What's your name"
Student in Picture: "My name is x" "I am X". etc

Non Verbal Response
Teacher/Therapist: "Who is this?"
Student in Picture: Points to self
Teacher/Therapist: "What's your name"
Student in Picture: Points to self, points to picture and self

Use of Communication Device
Teacher/Therapist: "Who is this?"
Student in Picture: "It's Me." "child's name" (chooses appropriate choice on board or device)
Teacher/Therapist: "What's your name"
Student in Picture: "My name is x" "I am X". etc (choose appropriate choice on board or device)

Cues/Modifications to Facilitate Responses

Provide only one choice – upgrade to more choices when picture discrimination is mastered

Provide mirror for students that cannot yet discriminate between self and representational images of self

Encourage responses – verbal, non-verbal and by using devices

Expand activity if students recognize themselves, but asking peers to discriminate and name each other.

Goodbye

Sit in front of the students and greet each child individually. Provide augmentative communication or choice board for students that need assistance responding. Encourage eye contact as appropriate. Fleeting eye contact is acceptable is the intent is to provide joint attention.

Direct Instruction Example
Teacher/Therapist: "It's time for us to end group time. "Goodbye Mrs. X!"
Teacher/Therapist: "Goodbye Mrs. X!" (or Hi puppet name)

Verbal Response
Teacher/Therapist: "It's time for us to end group time. Goodbye student x!"
Student X: "Goodbye Mrs. X. (or Hi puppet name)

Non Verbal Response
Teacher/Therapist: "It's time for us to end group time. Goodbye student x!"
Student X: Initiate eye contact, wave, smile in direction of teacher/therapist/puppet

Use of Communication Device
Teacher/Therapist: "It's time for us to end group time. Goodbye student x!"
Student X: Touch "Goodbye Mrs. X" on given choice board, communication device, Ipad, etc

Focus:
Trunk elongation
Overhead Extension
Underbody Flexion
Bilateral Use of Hands
Body Awareness
Prepositions (front, behind, over, under)

Materials:
Puppet (if using)
Playground ball or medium sized ball

Method:
In this activity, students will complete greeting sequence with appropriate follow through. Students with then participate in a ball activity requiring listening, imitating motor movements, and following directions.

Greeting

Sit in front of the students and greet each child individually. Provide augmentative communication or choice board for students that need assistance responding. Encourage eye contact as appropriate. Fleeting eye contact is acceptable is the intent is to provide joint attention.

Direct Instruction Example
Teacher/Therapist: "It's time for us to have group time. Hi Mrs. X!"
Teacher/Therapist: "Hi Mrs. X!" (or Hi puppet name)

Verbal Response
Teacher/Therapist: "It's time for us to have group time. Hi student x!"
Student X: "Hi Mrs. X. (or Hi puppet name)

Non Verbal Response
Teacher/Therapist: "It's time for us to have group time. Hi student x!"
Student X: Initiate eye contact, wave, smile in direction of teacher/therapist/puppet

Use of Communication Device
Teacher/Therapist: "It's time for us to have group time. Hi student x!"
Student X: Touch "Hi Mrs. X" on given choice board, communication device, Ipad, etc

Activity: Ball Exchange with Peers

Position students in a line in a sitting stance. Once all students are seated, demonstrate with another teacher how to pass the ball OVER head holding the ball with two hands and moving it with extended arms over to the teacher behind the instructor.

Be sure to encourage:
1. Trunk elongation
2. Arm extension
3. Holding ball with two hands
4. Maintaining hold on ball
5. Release ball when peer is ready to receive it

Provide hand over hand assistance as needed for students with poor motor planning or body awareness.

For language expansion and responses, talk about the experience:
Where are your arms? (Up)
Who is in front of you?
Who is behind you?
Who are you passing the ball to?
Who is giving you the ball?

Be sure to provide appropriate modifications for communication.

Goodbye
Sit in front of the students and greet each child individually. Provide augmentative communication or choice board for students that need assistance responding. Encourage eye contact as appropriate. Fleeting eye contact is acceptable is the intent is to provide joint attention.

Direct Instruction Example

Teacher/Therapist: "It's time for us to end group time. "Goodbye Mrs. X!"
Teacher/Therapist: "Goodbye Mrs. X!" (or Hi puppet name)

Verbal Response
Teacher/Therapist: "It's time for us to end group time. Goodbye student x!"
Student X: "Goodbye Mrs. X. (or Hi puppet name)

Non Verbal Response
Teacher/Therapist: "It's time for us to end group time. Goodbye student x!"
Student X: Initiate eye contact, wave, smile in direction of teacher/therapist/puppet

Use of Communication Device
Teacher/Therapist: "It's time for us to end group time. Goodbye student x!"
Student X: Touch "Goodbye Mrs. X" on given choice board, communication device, Ipad, etc

Focus:
Breath support
Trunk stability
Following directions
Stabilization with arm support

Materials:
Tissues
Ping Pong Balls

Method:

Greeting

Sit in front of the students and greet each child individually. Provide augmentative communication or choice board for students that need assistance responding. Encourage eye contact as appropriate. Fleeting eye contact is acceptable is the intent is to provide joint attention.

Direct Instruction Example
Teacher/Therapist: "It's time for us to have group time. Hi Mrs. X!"
Teacher/Therapist: "Hi Mrs. X!" (or Hi puppet name)

Verbal Response
Teacher/Therapist: "It's time for us to have group time. Hi student x!"
Student X: "Hi Mrs. X. (or Hi puppet name)

Non Verbal Response
Teacher/Therapist: "It's time for us to have group time. Hi student x!"
Student X: Initiate eye contact, wave, smile in direction of teacher/therapist/puppet

Use of Communication Device
Teacher/Therapist: "It's time for us to have group time. Hi student x!"
Student X: Touch "Hi Mrs. X" on given choice board, communication device, Ipad, etc

Sit at the table and ensure all students are sitting upright and in the correct position.

Demonstrate to the students how to inhale deeply (take a deep breath) and exhale (blow). Practice blowing – inhale/exhale.

Take a tissue from a box and hold it with two hands in front in the face. Inhale strongly and then blow the tissue to make it move.

Provide instruction on how to blow and make the tissue move. One by one provide a tissue for a student. Have them hold it with two hands, take in a large inhalation and blow hard enough to move the tissue.

Adaptation: Hold tissue for student.

Celebrate moving the tissue!

Activity: Blowing Ping Pong Balls

Have student remain seated at the table. Demonstrate to student how to position the ping-pong in front of the mouth and blow it across the table.

While seated, provide each student a ping-pong ball in front of the mouth and blow across the table. Ensure upright position. Celebrate moving the ball by moving.

Goodbye

Sit in front of the students and greet each child individually. Provide augmentative communication or choice board for students that need assistance responding. Encourage eye contact as appropriate. Fleeting eye contact is acceptable is the intent is to provide joint attention.

Direct Instruction Example
Teacher/Therapist: "It's time for us to end group time. "Goodbye Mrs. X!"
Teacher/Therapist: "Goodbye Mrs. X!" (or Hi puppet name)

Verbal Response
Teacher/Therapist: "It's time for us to end group time. Goodbye student x!"

Student X: "Goodbye Mrs. X. (or Hi puppet name)

Non Verbal Response
Teacher/Therapist: "It's time for us to end group time. Goodbye student x!"
Student X: Initiate eye contact, wave, smile in direction of teacher/therapist/puppet

Use of Communication Device
Teacher/Therapist: "It's time for us to end group time. Goodbye student x!"
Student X: Touch "Goodbye Mrs. X" on given choice board, communication device, Ipad, etc.

Focus:
Breath support
Trunk stability
Following directions
Bilateral Integration
Eye hand coordination

Materials:
Bubbles
Cotton Balls
Straw

Method:

Greeting

Sit in front of the students and greet each child individually. Provide augmentative communication or choice board for students that need assistance responding. Encourage eye contact as appropriate. Fleeting eye contact is acceptable is the intent is to provide joint attention.

Direct Instruction Example
Teacher/Therapist: "It's time for us to have group time. Hi Mrs. X!"
Teacher/Therapist: "Hi Mrs. X!" (or Hi puppet name)

Verbal Response
Teacher/Therapist: "It's time for us to have group time. Hi student x!"
Student X: "Hi Mrs. X. (or Hi puppet name)

Non Verbal Response
Teacher/Therapist: "It's time for us to have group time. Hi student x!"
Student X: Initiate eye contact, wave, smile in direction of teacher/therapist/puppet

Use of Communication Device
Teacher/Therapist: "It's time for us to have group time. Hi student x!"
Student X: Touch "Hi Mrs. X" on given choice board, communication device, Ipad, etc

Activity: Bubbles

While seated on the floor, have the students observe you blowing bubbles. Provide instruction to WAIT (don't pop or get up to play with bubbles). Encourage the concept of wait and watch the bubbles.

One by one provide the students the opportunity to use two hands to pop the bubbles once an adult has blown them. Practice using two hands coming together to pop the bubbles. Encourage students to wait for his/her turn.

After each student has popped bubbles with two hands, turn the focus to blowing bubbles with a large inhalation and exhalation. With each student, practice holding the bubble wand and blowing the bubble.

Adaptation: Hold the bubble wand at the mouth and prompting blowing from behind the student (so they "feel" blowing).

Activity: Cotton Balls

Place students in the chairs at the table. Ensure that students are sitting upright and positioned properly to inhale and exhale effectively.

Place a cotton ball on the table. Demonstrate to each student how to inhale and exhale in a manner that moves the cotton ball across the table.

One at a time, provide a student with a cotton ball and have them blow it across the table.

Modification: Use straw when exhaling

Additional blowing tasks:
  Blowing party blowers
  Blowing whistles
  Blowing feathers
  Blowing leaves

Goodbye

Sit in front of the students and greet each child individually. Provide augmentative communication or choice board for students that need assistance responding. Encourage eye contact as appropriate. Fleeting eye contact is acceptable is the intent is to provide joint attention.

Direct Instruction Example
Teacher/Therapist: "It's time for us to end group time. "Goodbye Mrs. X!"
Teacher/Therapist: "Goodbye Mrs. X!" (or Hi puppet name)

Verbal Response
Teacher/Therapist: "It's time for us to end group time. Goodbye student x!"
Student X: "Goodbye Mrs. X. (or Hi puppet name)

Non Verbal Response
Teacher/Therapist: "It's time for us to end group time. Goodbye student x!"
Student X: Initiate eye contact, wave, smile in direction of teacher/therapist/puppet

Use of Communication Device
Teacher/Therapist: "It's time for us to end group time. Goodbye student x!"
Student X: Touch "Goodbye Mrs. X" on given choice board, communication device, Ipad, etc

Focus:
Breath support
Trunk stability
Following directions

Materials:
None

Method:

Greeting

Sit in front of the students and greet each child individually. Provide augmentative communication or choice board for students that need assistance responding. Encourage eye contact as appropriate. Fleeting eye contact is acceptable is the intent is to provide joint attention.

Direct Instruction Example
Teacher/Therapist: "It's time for us to have group time. Hi Mrs. X!"
Teacher/Therapist: "Hi Mrs. X!" (or Hi puppet name)

Verbal Response
Teacher/Therapist: "It's time for us to have group time. Hi student x!"
Student X: "Hi Mrs. X. (or Hi puppet name)

Non Verbal Response
Teacher/Therapist: "It's time for us to have group time. Hi student x!"
Student X: Initiate eye contact, wave, smile in direction of teacher/therapist/puppet

Use of Communication Device
Teacher/Therapist: "It's time for us to have group time. Hi student x!"
Student X: Touch "Hi Mrs. X" on given choice board, communication device, Ipad, etc

Provide an example to students on how to play London Bridge. Partner with an adult and extend arms overhead while holding hands. Have another adult going around the "bridge" and sing the song.
Two adults hold hands to create a bridge and individually have students go through the bridge while group sings the song.

Advancement: Have two students create a bridge and have another student pass through bridge while group sings the song.

Activity: Row Your Boat

Demonstrate how to sit on the floor with another adult. Put feet together in a V-shape position and hold hands. Begin to sing row a boat and pull each other reciprocally.

Provide individual instruction of the process by having each student pair up with the adult. Sing row your boat with each student and encourage him or her to pull and push as the song is sung.

Advancement: Have students paired up and independently complete row your boat task with peer.

Goodbye
Sit in front of the students and greet each child individually. Provide augmentative communication or choice board for students that need assistance responding. Encourage eye contact as appropriate. Fleeting eye contact is acceptable is the intent is to provide joint attention.

Direct Instruction Example
Teacher/Therapist: "It's time for us to end group time. "Goodbye Mrs. X!"
Teacher/Therapist: "Goodbye Mrs. X!" (or Hi puppet name)

Verbal Response
Teacher/Therapist: "It's time for us to end group time. Goodbye student x!"
Student X: "Goodbye Mrs. X. (or Hi puppet name)

Non Verbal Response

Teacher/Therapist: "It's time for us to end group time. Goodbye student x!"
Student X: Initiate eye contact, wave, smile in direction of teacher/therapist/puppet

Use of Communication Device
Teacher/Therapist: "It's time for us to end group time. Goodbye student x!"
Student X: Touch "Goodbye Mrs. X" on given choice board, communication device, Ipad, etc

Focus:
Breath support
Trunk stability
Following directions
Maintaining Strong Hold/Holding tight
Trunk elongation
Heavy work/sensory input

Materials:
Scooterboard
Hula Hoop

Method:

Greeting

Sit in front of the students and greet each child individually. Provide augmentative communication or choice board for students that need assistance responding. Encourage eye contact as appropriate. Fleeting eye contact is acceptable is the intent is to provide joint attention.

Direct Instruction Example
Teacher/Therapist: "It's time for us to have group time. Hi Mrs. X!"
Teacher/Therapist: "Hi Mrs. X!" (or Hi puppet name)

Verbal Response
Teacher/Therapist: "It's time for us to have group time. Hi student x!"
Student X: "Hi Mrs. X. (or Hi puppet name)

Non Verbal Response
Teacher/Therapist: "It's time for us to have group time. Hi student x!"
Student X: Initiate eye contact, wave, smile in direction of teacher/therapist/puppet

Use of Communication Device
Teacher/Therapist: "It's time for us to have group time. Hi student x!"
Student X: Touch "Hi Mrs. X" on given choice board, communication device, Ipad, etc

Show each student how to lie prone on the scooterboard. Extend arms and legs, keep neck extended and head erect while lying prone. Talk to student about your body's position.

Have another adult pull you on the scooterboard in the classroom or hallway while you remain prone and extended. Keep your feet up (remind students of this) and keep your grip tight on the hula hoop (remind students of this)

Provide the experience to each student. Ensure each student:
1. Extend arms and legs
2. Maintain hold on hula hoop
3. Keep head and neck extended and erect
4. Keep legs up

Goodbye

Sit in front of the students and greet each child individually. Provide augmentative communication or choice board for students that need assistance responding. Encourage eye contact as appropriate. Fleeting eye contact is acceptable is the intent is to provide joint attention.

Direct Instruction Example
Teacher/Therapist: "It's time for us to end group time. "Goodbye Mrs. X!"
Teacher/Therapist: "Goodbye Mrs. X!" (or Hi puppet name)

Verbal Response
Teacher/Therapist: "It's time for us to end group time. Goodbye student x!"
Student X: "Goodbye Mrs. X. (or Hi puppet name)

Non Verbal Response
Teacher/Therapist: "It's time for us to end group time. Goodbye student x!"
Student X: Initiate eye contact, wave, smile in direction of teacher/therapist/puppet

Use of Communication Device
Teacher/Therapist: "It's time for us to end group time. Goodbye student x!"
Student X: Touch "Goodbye Mrs. X" on given choice board, communication device, Ipad, etc

Focus:
Breath support
Trunk stability
Following directions

Materials:
Broomstick
Pinwheels

Methods

Greeting

Sit in front of the students and greet each child individually. Provide augmentative communication or choice board for students that need assistance responding. Encourage eye contact as appropriate. Fleeting eye contact is acceptable is the intent is to provide joint attention.

Direct Instruction Example
Teacher/Therapist: "It's time for us to have group time. Hi Mrs. X!"
Teacher/Therapist: "Hi Mrs. X!" (or Hi puppet name)

Verbal Response
Teacher/Therapist: "It's time for us to have group time. Hi student x!"
Student X: "Hi Mrs. X. (or Hi puppet name)

Non Verbal Response
Teacher/Therapist: "It's time for us to have group time. Hi student x!"
Student X: Initiate eye contact, wave, smile in direction of teacher/therapist/puppet

Use of Communication Device
Teacher/Therapist: "It's time for us to have group time. Hi student x!"
Student X: Touch "Hi Mrs. X" on given choice board, communication device, Ipad, etc

Talk about monkeys with students.

What do monkeys say?
What do monkeys do?

Explain that each student will pretend being a monkey swinging from a tree. Demonstrate how the broomstick will be the tree and how the students will hold tight to "swing".

With adult assistance with the other end of the broomstick, lower the broomstick to allow the student to grab it. Reinforce the feeling of "holding tight" by placing your hands over the child's and squeezing it slightly to teacher "tight". Once child understands holding on, life him/her up and count how long he/she can maintain hold while swinging. Attempt to count to ten, but adjust as necessary for student needs.

Activity: Pinwheel Play

While seated in chairs, show students the pinwheel and demonstrate how blowing moves the pinwheel.

Provide each student a turn blowing the pinwheel. Hold the pinwheel in front of the student so he/she can focus on just blowing.

Advancement: Have the student sit upright, hold the pinwheel and while blowing.

Goodbye
Sit in front of the students and greet each child individually. Provide augmentative communication or choice board for students that need assistance responding. Encourage eye contact as appropriate. Fleeting eye contact is acceptable is the intent is to provide joint attention.

Direct Instruction Example
Teacher/Therapist: "It's time for us to end group time. "Goodbye Mrs. X!"
Teacher/Therapist: "Goodbye Mrs. X!" (or Hi puppet name)

Verbal Response
Teacher/Therapist: "It's time for us to end group time. Goodbye student x!"

Student X: "Goodbye Mrs. X. (or Hi puppet name)

Non Verbal Response
Teacher/Therapist: "It's time for us to end group time. Goodbye student x!"
Student X: Initiate eye contact, wave, smile in direction of teacher/therapist/puppet

Use of Communication Device
Teacher/Therapist: "It's time for us to end group time. Goodbye student x!"
Student X: Touch "Goodbye Mrs. X" on given choice board, communication device, Ipad, etc.

Week 8

Focus:
Breath support
Trunk stability
Following directions

Materials:
Cube Chair

Method:

Greeting

Sit in front of the students and greet each child individually. Provide augmentative communication or choice board for students that need assistance responding. Encourage eye contact as appropriate. Fleeting eye contact is acceptable is the intent is to provide joint attention.

Direct Instruction Example
Teacher/Therapist: "It's time for us to have group time. Hi Mrs. X!"
Teacher/Therapist: "Hi Mrs. X!" (or Hi puppet name)

Verbal Response
Teacher/Therapist: "It's time for us to have group time. Hi student x!"
Student X: "Hi Mrs. X. (or Hi puppet name)

Non Verbal Response
Teacher/Therapist: "It's time for us to have group time. Hi student x!"
Student X: Initiate eye contact, wave, smile in direction of teacher/therapist/puppet

Use of Communication Device
Teacher/Therapist: "It's time for us to have group time. Hi student x!"
Student X: Touch "Hi Mrs. X" on given choice board, communication device, Ipad, etc

Activity: Cube Running

Locate cube chairs for this activity. There are two ways to race with the cube chair 1) in tall kneel or 2) standing.

In tall kneel, push the cube chair with arms extended out in front of them while pushing the chair.

In standing, push the cube chair with arms extended and the chair in front of them.

Assist students with task with physical cues or stability if needed. Monitor students for assistance with task.

To ensure students know how to complete the task, have each student race with the cube chair individually before racing a peer.

Goodbye

 Sit in front of the students and greet each child individually. Provide augmentative communication or choice board for students that need assistance responding. Encourage eye contact as appropriate. Fleeting eye contact is acceptable is the intent is to provide joint attention.

Direct Instruction Example
Teacher/Therapist: "It's time for us to end group time. "Goodbye Mrs. X!"
Teacher/Therapist: "Goodbye Mrs. X!" (or Hi puppet name)

Verbal Response
Teacher/Therapist: "It's time for us to end group time. Goodbye student x!"
Student X: "Goodbye Mrs. X. (or Hi puppet name)

Non Verbal Response
Teacher/Therapist: "It's time for us to end group time. Goodbye student x!"
Student X: Initiate eye contact, wave, smile in direction of teacher/therapist/puppet

Use of Communication Device
Teacher/Therapist: "It's time for us to end group time. Goodbye student x!"
Student X: Touch "Goodbye Mrs. X" on given choice board, communication device, Ipad, etc

Focus:
Wrist rotation
In hand manipulation
Pincer grasp

Materials:
Wind up toys
Baby jar with lids/or various jar with lids
M&M or desirable candy of choice

Method:

Greeting

Sit in front of the students and greet each child individually. Provide augmentative communication or choice board for students that need assistance responding. Encourage eye contact as appropriate. Fleeting eye contact is acceptable is the intent is to provide joint attention.

Direct Instruction Example
Teacher/Therapist: "It's time for us to have group time. Hi Mrs. X!"
Teacher/Therapist: "Hi Mrs. X!" (or Hi puppet name)

Verbal Response
Teacher/Therapist: "It's time for us to have group time. Hi student x!"
Student X: "Hi Mrs. X. (or Hi puppet name)

Non Verbal Response
Teacher/Therapist: "It's time for us to have group time. Hi student x!"
Student X: Initiate eye contact, wave, smile in direction of teacher/therapist/puppet

Use of Communication Device
Teacher/Therapist: "It's time for us to have group time. Hi student x!"
Student X: Touch "Hi Mrs. X" on given choice board, communication device, Ipad, etc

Activity: Wind Up Toy Twisting

While seated at the table, show the students the various wind up toys and how you twist them up to make them move. Discuss how to use the thumb, index finger and middle finger to twist.

Provide each student with a wind up toy and practice using a pincer grasp to wind it up. Switch toys to continue practicing with task.

Activity: Baby Jar Twisting

Put a candy or M&M in each jar and close the lid. Adjust for student needs, especially in regards to choking hazards. Choose an alternative motivator if candy is unsafe.

Give a jar to each student and request him/her to open the jar. Encourage shoulder stability and wrist rotation during task.

Add more M&Ms for continued practice.

Goodbye

Sit in front of the students and greet each child individually. Provide augmentative communication or choice board for students that need assistance responding. Encourage eye contact as appropriate. Fleeting eye contact is acceptable is the intent is to provide joint attention.

Direct Instruction Example
Teacher/Therapist: "It's time for us to end group time. "Goodbye Mrs. X!"
Teacher/Therapist: "Goodbye Mrs. X!" (or Hi puppet name)

Verbal Response
Teacher/Therapist: "It's time for us to end group time. Goodbye student x!"
Student X: "Goodbye Mrs. X. (or Hi puppet name)

Non Verbal Response
Teacher/Therapist: "It's time for us to end group time. Goodbye student x!"
Student X: Initiate eye contact, wave, smile in direction of teacher/therapist/puppet

Use of Communication Device
Teacher/Therapist: "It's time for us to end group time. Goodbye student x!"

Student X: Touch "Goodbye Mrs. X" on given choice board, communication device, Ipad, etc

Focus:
Wrist rotation
In hand rotation

Materials:
Slinky
Rain Sticks

Method:

Greeting

Sit in front of the students and greet each child individually. Provide augmentative communication or choice board for students that need assistance responding. Encourage eye contact as appropriate. Fleeting eye contact is acceptable is the intent is to provide joint attention.

Direct Instruction Example
Teacher/Therapist: "It's time for us to have group time. Hi Mrs. X!"
Teacher/Therapist: "Hi Mrs. X!" (or Hi puppet name)

Verbal Response
Teacher/Therapist: "It's time for us to have group time. Hi student x!"
Student X: "Hi Mrs. X. (or Hi puppet name)

Non Verbal Response
Teacher/Therapist: "It's time for us to have group time. Hi student x!"
Student X: Initiate eye contact, wave, smile in direction of teacher/therapist/puppet

Use of Communication Device
Teacher/Therapist: "It's time for us to have group time. Hi student x!"
Student X: Touch "Hi Mrs. X" on given choice board, communication device, Ipad, etc

Activity: Slinky

Place slinky in hand. Encourage moving the hand up and down to move the slinky. Practice control to keep the slinky in the hand and maintaining movement and balance.

Activity: Rain Stick

Provide student a rain stick. Encourage wrist rotation to flip the rain stick to make noise.

Goodbye

Sit in front of the students and greet each child individually. Provide augmentative communication or choice board for students that need assistance responding. Encourage eye contact as appropriate. Fleeting eye contact is acceptable is the intent is to provide joint attention.

Direct Instruction Example
Teacher/Therapist: "It's time for us to end group time. "Goodbye Mrs. X!"
Teacher/Therapist: "Goodbye Mrs. X!" (or Hi puppet name)

Verbal Response
Teacher/Therapist: "It's time for us to end group time. Goodbye student x!"
Student X: "Goodbye Mrs. X. (or Hi puppet name)

Non Verbal Response
Teacher/Therapist: "It's time for us to end group time. Goodbye student x!"
Student X: Initiate eye contact, wave, smile in direction of teacher/therapist/puppet

Use of Communication Device
Teacher/Therapist: "It's time for us to end group time. Goodbye student x!"
Student X: Touch "Goodbye Mrs. X" on given choice board, communication device, Ipad, etc

Focus:
Wrist Rotation
In hand manipulation
Visual Discrimination
Visual Scanning
Visual Memory

Materials:
Cups with pictures of choice under them (with matches not under cup)
Pair of pictures of choice
(Pictures may be related to theme)

Method:

Greeting

Sit in front of the students and greet each child individually. Provide augmentative communication or choice board for students that need assistance responding. Encourage eye contact as appropriate. Fleeting eye contact is acceptable is the intent is to provide joint attention.

Direct Instruction Example
Teacher/Therapist: "It's time for us to have group time. Hi Mrs. X!"
Teacher/Therapist: "Hi Mrs. X!" (or Hi puppet name)

Verbal Response
Teacher/Therapist: "It's time for us to have group time. Hi student x!"
Student X: "Hi Mrs. X. (or Hi puppet name)

Non Verbal Response
Teacher/Therapist: "It's time for us to have group time. Hi student x!"
Student X: Initiate eye contact, wave, smile in direction of teacher/therapist/puppet

Use of Communication Device
Teacher/Therapist: "It's time for us to have group time. Hi student x!"
Student X: Touch "Hi Mrs. X" on given choice board, communication device, Ipad, etc

Activity: Cup Flip

Put pictures on the inside of the cups (bottom of cup). Place various pictures on the floor that match. Adjust the choices for student skill – decrease the number of pictures to discriminate from based on student need.

Provide choices for the cups, start with two turned over cups. Ask student to turn over cup and look at picture. Encourage the student to communicate what they see. Use adaptations to communicate. Turn the cup back over and ask student to find the matching picture on floor. Continue for each student, adapting task for student skill regarding:
Visual discrimination skills (A student at Level 3 PECS needs only one cup and one match, for example)

Activity: Picture Matching

Place pictures on floor and hold matches in the your hand. Show the student a picture in your hand. In four point, have the student turn a picture over from the floor. Have the student communicate what picture is turned over and if it matches. If no, continue the process until the correct match is found.

Goodbye

Sit in front of the students and greet each child individually. Provide augmentative communication or choice board for students that need assistance responding. Encourage eye contact as appropriate. Fleeting eye contact is acceptable is the intent is to provide joint attention.

Direct Instruction Example
Teacher/Therapist: "It's time for us to end group time. "Goodbye Mrs. X!"
Teacher/Therapist: "Goodbye Mrs. X!" (or Hi puppet name)

Verbal Response
Teacher/Therapist: "It's time for us to end group time. Goodbye student x!"
Student X: "Goodbye Mrs. X. (or Hi puppet name)

Non Verbal Response
Teacher/Therapist: "It's time for us to end group time. Goodbye student x!"
Student X: Initiate eye contact, wave, smile in direction of teacher/therapist/puppet

Use of Communication Device
Teacher/Therapist: "It's time for us to end group time. Goodbye student x!"
Student X: Touch "Goodbye Mrs. X" on given choice board, communication device, Ipad, etc

Week 12

Focus:
In hand manipulation
Fine motor control
Eye hand coordination
Muscle gradation

Materials:
Circle shaped cereal
Pipe Cleaner
Yarn

Method:

Greeting

Sit in front of the students and greet each child individually. Provide augmentative communication or choice board for students that need assistance responding. Encourage eye contact as appropriate. Fleeting eye contact is acceptable is the intent is to provide joint attention.

Direct Instruction Example
Teacher/Therapist: "It's time for us to have group time. Hi Mrs. X!"
Teacher/Therapist: "Hi Mrs. X!" (or Hi puppet name)

Verbal Response
Teacher/Therapist: "It's time for us to have group time. Hi student x!"
Student X: "Hi Mrs. X. (or Hi puppet name)

Non-Verbal Response
Teacher/Therapist: "It's time for us to have group time. Hi student x!"
Student X: Initiate eye contact, wave, smile in direction of teacher/therapist/puppet

Use of Communication Device
Teacher/Therapist: "It's time for us to have group time. Hi student x!"
Student X: Touch "Hi Mrs. X" on given choice board, communication device, Ipad, etc.

Activity: Cereal Necklace

Before the activity, make a tie at the end of a pipecleaner (to stop cereal) and pull three cereal pieces to demonstrate how they look on the pipecleaner. Demonstrate how to look for the hole and pull the pipecleaner through the cereal. Provide enough cereal to complete a bracelet.

Activity: Cereal Necklace (yarn)

Same as above except use yarn.

Goodbye

Sit in front of the students and greet each child individually. Provide augmentative communication or choice board for students that need assistance responding. Encourage eye contact as appropriate. Fleeting eye contact is acceptable is the intent is to provide joint attention.

Direct Instruction Example
Teacher/Therapist: "It's time for us to end group time. "Goodbye Mrs. X!"
Teacher/Therapist: "Goodbye Mrs. X!" (or Hi puppet name)

Verbal Response
Teacher/Therapist: "It's time for us to end group time. Goodbye student x!"
Student X: "Goodbye Mrs. X. (or Hi puppet name)

Non Verbal Response
Teacher/Therapist: "It's time for us to end group time. Goodbye student x!"
Student X: Initiate eye contact, wave, smile in direction of teacher/therapist/puppet

Use of Communication Device
Teacher/Therapist: "It's time for us to end group time. Goodbye student x!"
Student X: Touch "Goodbye Mrs. X" on given choice board, communication device, Ipad, etc.

Focus:
In hand manipulation
Fine motor control
Eye hand coordination
Muscle gradation

Materials:
Puppet
Dry Noodles

Method:

Greeting

Sit in front of the students and greet each child individually. Provide augmentative communication or choice board for students that need assistance responding. Encourage eye contact as appropriate. Fleeting eye contact is acceptable is the intent is to provide joint attention.

Direct Instruction Example
Teacher/Therapist: "It's time for us to have group time. Hi Mrs. X!"
Teacher/Therapist: "Hi Mrs. X!" (or Hi puppet name)

Verbal Response
Teacher/Therapist: "It's time for us to have group time. Hi student x!"
Student X: "Hi Mrs. X. (or Hi puppet name)

Non Verbal Response
Teacher/Therapist: "It's time for us to have group time. Hi student x!"
Student X: Initiate eye contact, wave, smile in direction of teacher/therapist/puppet

Use of Communication Device
Teacher/Therapist: "It's time for us to have group time. Hi student x!"
Student X: Touch "Hi Mrs. X" on given choice board, communication device, Ipad, etc.

Provide a student with a puppet. Demonstrate how to do the following with the puppet:

1. Put puppet on
2. Open puppet mouth
3. Close puppet mouth
4. Make puppet dance
5. Make puppet bow
6. Make puppet talk, sing
7. Make puppet lie on floor
8. Make puppet roll over
9. Make puppet wake up

With puppet positioned on teacher hand, have students sit in front of the puppet. Discuss how to "feed" the puppet. Put dried macaroni on the table and ask the student to use a pincer grasp to pick up one macaroni. Provide the following:

1. Ask the puppet if he wants something to eat.
2. Use communication devices if needed to facilitate choices
3. When the response is yes, then have the student prompt the puppet to open his mouth.
4. Use communication devices if needed to request open
5. Once mouth is open, use pincer grasping pattern to place the macaroni into the puppet's mouth
6. Ask the puppet if he wants more, continue feeding using pincer grasping pattern to obtain macaroni.

Advancement: Have a student play the role of puppet and another play the role of feeder

Sit in front of the students and greet each child individually. Provide augmentative communication or choice board for students that need assistance responding. Encourage eye contact as appropriate. Fleeting eye contact is acceptable is the intent is to provide joint attention.

Direct Instruction Example
Teacher/Therapist: "It's time for us to end group time. "Goodbye Mrs. X!"
Teacher/Therapist: "Goodbye Mrs. X!" (or Hi puppet name)

Verbal Response
Teacher/Therapist: "It's time for us to end group time. Goodbye student x!"
Student X: "Goodbye Mrs. X. (or Hi puppet name)

Non Verbal Response
Teacher/Therapist: "It's time for us to end group time. Goodbye student x!"
Student X: Initiate eye contact, wave, smile in direction of teacher/therapist/puppet

Use of Communication Device
Teacher/Therapist: "It's time for us to end group time. Goodbye student x!"
Student X: Touch "Goodbye Mrs. X" on given choice board, communication device, Ipad, etc.

Week 14

Focus:
In hand manipulation
Fine motor control
Eye hand coordination
Muscle gradation

Materials:
Clothespins
Coffee Can
Tweezers
Strawberry Huller
Small pom pom/cotton

Method:

Greeting

Sit in front of the students and greet each child individually. Provide augmentative communication or choice board for students that need assistance responding. Encourage eye contact as appropriate. Fleeting eye contact is acceptable is the intent is to provide joint attention.

Direct Instruction Example
Teacher/Therapist: "It's time for us to have group time. Hi Mrs. X!"
Teacher/Therapist: "Hi Mrs. X!" (or Hi puppet name)

Verbal Response
Teacher/Therapist: "It's time for us to have group time. Hi student x!"
Student X: "Hi Mrs. X. (or Hi puppet name)

Non Verbal Response
Teacher/Therapist: "It's time for us to have group time. Hi student x!"
Student X: Initiate eye contact, wave, smile in direction of teacher/therapist/puppet

Use of Communication Device
Teacher/Therapist: "It's time for us to have group time. Hi student x!"

Student X: Touch "Hi Mrs. X" on given choice board, communication device, Ipad, etc.

Activity: Clothespin Pinching

Prior to the start of the activity, have all the clothespins on the top of a coffee can. Have the students use a pincer grasp to remove the clothespins from the can and release them into the can.

Advancement: Use pincer grasp to place the clothespins on the top of the coffee can.

Activity: Tweezer Pickup

Prior to the start of activity, place the small items (cotton, koosh) on the table in a scattered about.
Ask the students to use tweezers to pick up the items and place them in the can.

Goodbye

Sit in front of the students and greet each child individually. Provide augmentative communication or choice board for students that need assistance responding. Encourage eye contact as appropriate. Fleeting eye contact is acceptable is the intent is to provide joint attention.

Direct Instruction Example
Teacher/Therapist: "It's time for us to end group time. "Goodbye Mrs. X!"
Teacher/Therapist: "Goodbye Mrs. X!" (or Hi puppet name)

Verbal Response
Teacher/Therapist: "It's time for us to end group time. Goodbye student x!"
Student X: "Goodbye Mrs. X. (or Hi puppet name)

Non Verbal Response
Teacher/Therapist: "It's time for us to end group time. Goodbye student x!"
Student X: Initiate eye contact, wave, smile in direction of teacher/therapist/puppet

Use of Communication Device
Teacher/Therapist: "It's time for us to end group time. Goodbye student x!"
Student X: Touch "Goodbye Mrs. X" on given choice board, communication device, Ipad, etc.

Focus:
In hand manipulation
Fine motor control
Eye hand coordination
Muscle gradation

Materials:
Theraputty
Pennies
Hairbeads
Coffee Can with a slit made for pennies

Method:

Greeting

Sit in front of the students and greet each child individually. Provide augmentative communication or choice board for students that need assistance responding. Encourage eye contact as appropriate. Fleeting eye contact is acceptable is the intent is to provide joint attention.

Direct Instruction Example
Teacher/Therapist: "It's time for us to have group time. Hi Mrs. X!"
Teacher/Therapist: "Hi Mrs. X!" (or Hi puppet name)

Verbal Response
Teacher/Therapist: "It's time for us to have group time. Hi student x!"
Student X: "Hi Mrs. X. (or Hi puppet name)

Non Verbal Response
Teacher/Therapist: "It's time for us to have group time. Hi student x!"
Student X: Initiate eye contact, wave, smile in direction of teacher/therapist/puppet

Use of Communication Device
Teacher/Therapist: "It's time for us to have group time. Hi student x!"
Student X: Touch "Hi Mrs. X" on given choice board, communication device, Ipad, etc.

Activity: Theraputty (Pennies, Hairbeads)

Prior to activity place pennies or hairbeads into theraputty.
Have students manipulate the theraputty to remove pennies and hairbeads.

Activity: Pennies in Can

Place pennies in a pile on the non-dominant side of the student. Have the student pick up the pennies using a pincer grasping pattern and put them in the can.

Goodbye

Sit in front of the students and greet each child individually. Provide augmentative communication or choice board for students that need assistance responding. Encourage eye contact as appropriate. Fleeting eye contact is acceptable is the intent is to provide joint attention.

Direct Instruction Example
Teacher/Therapist: "It's time for us to end group time. "Goodbye Mrs. X!"
Teacher/Therapist: "Goodbye Mrs. X!" (or Hi puppet name)

Verbal Response
Teacher/Therapist: "It's time for us to end group time. Goodbye student x!"
Student X: "Goodbye Mrs. X. (or Hi puppet name)

Non Verbal Response
Teacher/Therapist: "It's time for us to end group time. Goodbye student x!"
Student X: Initiate eye contact, wave, smile in direction of teacher/therapist/puppet

Use of Communication Device
Teacher/Therapist: "It's time for us to end group time. Goodbye student x!"
Student X: Touch "Goodbye Mrs. X" on given choice board, communication device, Ipad, etc.

Focus:
In hand manipulation
Fine motor control
Eye hand coordination
Muscle gradation

Materials:
Shaving Cream
Towels
Plastic baby doll

Method:

Greeting

Sit in front of the students and greet each child individually. Provide augmentative communication or choice board for students that need assistance responding. Encourage eye contact as appropriate. Fleeting eye contact is acceptable is the intent is to provide joint attention.

Direct Instruction Example
Teacher/Therapist: "It's time for us to have group time. Hi Mrs. X!"
Teacher/Therapist: "Hi Mrs. X!" (or Hi puppet name)

Verbal Response
Teacher/Therapist: "It's time for us to have group time. Hi student x!"
Student X: "Hi Mrs. X. (or Hi puppet name)

Non Verbal Response
Teacher/Therapist: "It's time for us to have group time. Hi student x!"
Student X: Initiate eye contact, wave, smile in direction of teacher/therapist/puppet

Use of Communication Device
Teacher/Therapist: "It's time for us to have group time. Hi student x!"
Student X: Touch "Hi Mrs. X" on given choice board, communication device, Ipad, etc.

Activity: Washing Baby

Provide each student with a baby doll. Squirt shaving cream (or alternative cleaning material, foam soap) all over baby doll. Have the student clean the baby doll using paper towels.

Talk about the following:
Is the baby clean or dirty?
Where are you cleaning?
Identify body parts as they are being cleaned.

Activity: Washing Chair

Do the same as above, but "clean" a plastic chair

Goodbye

 Sit in front of the students and greet each child individually. Provide augmentative communication or choice board for students that need assistance responding. Encourage eye contact as appropriate. Fleeting eye contact is acceptable is the intent is to provide joint attention.

Direct Instruction Example
Teacher/Therapist: "It's time for us to end group time. "Goodbye Mrs. X!"
Teacher/Therapist: "Goodbye Mrs. X!" (or Hi puppet name)

Verbal Response
Teacher/Therapist: "It's time for us to end group time. Goodbye student x!"
Student X: "Goodbye Mrs. X. (or Hi puppet name)

Non Verbal Response
Teacher/Therapist: "It's time for us to end group time. Goodbye student x!"
Student X: Initiate eye contact, wave, smile in direction of teacher/therapist/puppet

Use of Communication Device
Teacher/Therapist: "It's time for us to end group time. Goodbye student x!"
Student X: Touch "Goodbye Mrs. X" on given choice board, communication device, Ipad, etc.

Focus:
In hand manipulation
Fine motor control
Eye hand coordination
Muscle gradation

Materials:
Two buckets
6 sponges
Water in one bucket

Method:

Greeting

Sit in front of the students and greet each child individually. Provide augmentative communication or choice board for students that need assistance responding. Encourage eye contact as appropriate. Fleeting eye contact is acceptable is the intent is to provide joint attention.

Direct Instruction Example
Teacher/Therapist: "It's time for us to have group time. Hi Mrs. X!"
Teacher/Therapist: "Hi Mrs. X!" (or Hi puppet name)

Verbal Response
Teacher/Therapist: "It's time for us to have group time. Hi student x!"
Student X: "Hi Mrs. X. (or Hi puppet name)

Non Verbal Response
Teacher/Therapist: "It's time for us to have group time. Hi student x!"
Student X: Initiate eye contact, wave, smile in direction of teacher/therapist/puppet

Use of Communication Device
Teacher/Therapist: "It's time for us to have group time. Hi student x!"
Student X: Touch "Hi Mrs. X" on given choice board, communication device, Ipad, etc.

Activity: Water Bucket

Prior to the activity, put water in the one of the buckets. Place the water filled bucket about ten feet away from the empty bucket. Place sponges in the water bucket and all the water to soak it.

Teach students to transfer six sponges (one by one) from the water bucket to the dry bucket. Have the student squeeze the sponge in the dry bucket to fill it. Encourage students to hold the sponge gently and not to prematurely squeeze the sponge.

Goodbye

Sit in front of the students and greet each child individually. Provide augmentative communication or choice board for students that need assistance responding. Encourage eye contact as appropriate. Fleeting eye contact is acceptable is the intent is to provide joint attention.

Direct Instruction Example
Teacher/Therapist: "It's time for us to end group time. "Goodbye Mrs. X!"
Teacher/Therapist: "Goodbye Mrs. X!" (or Hi puppet name)

Verbal Response
Teacher/Therapist: "It's time for us to end group time. Goodbye student x!"
Student X: "Goodbye Mrs. X. (or Hi puppet name)

Non Verbal Response
Teacher/Therapist: "It's time for us to end group time. Goodbye student x!"
Student X: Initiate eye contact, wave, smile in direction of teacher/therapist/puppet

Use of Communication Device
Teacher/Therapist: "It's time for us to end group time. Goodbye student x!"
Student X: Touch "Goodbye Mrs. X" on given choice board, communication device, Ipad, etc.

Focus:
Gross motor skills
Follow directions
Extension arms

Materials:
Parachute
Stuffed Animal

Method:

Greeting

Sit in front of the students and greet each child individually. Provide augmentative communication or choice board for students that need assistance responding. Encourage eye contact as appropriate. Fleeting eye contact is acceptable is the intent is to provide joint attention.

Direct Instruction Example
Teacher/Therapist: "It's time for us to have group time. Hi Mrs. X!"
Teacher/Therapist: "Hi Mrs. X!" (or Hi puppet name)

Verbal Response
Teacher/Therapist: "It's time for us to have group time. Hi student x!"
Student X: "Hi Mrs. X. (or Hi puppet name)

Non Verbal Response
Teacher/Therapist: "It's time for us to have group time. Hi student x!"
Student X: Initiate eye contact, wave, smile in direction of teacher/therapist/puppet

Use of Communication Device
Teacher/Therapist: "It's time for us to have group time. Hi student x!"
Student X: Touch "Hi Mrs. X" on given choice board, communication device, Ipad, etc.

Activity: Parachute Play
Provide directions on rules related to parachute play

1. Wait
2. No running
3. No stepping on parachute
4. No getting under parachute unless directed
5. LISTEN

Assist each child in holding the parachute loop and show how to maintain position to hold the loop. Begin lifting the parachute up and down to make the parachute "shake". Have the students all "shake" the parachute.

Review the concepts of "slow shake" (moving up and down slowly) and "fast shake" (moving up and down very fast)

Introduce the concepts of "up" and "down".

Place stuffed animal in the middle and watch him bounce around as you direct the students to "shake" – practice "slow", "fast", "up", "down".

Introduce walking around in a circle while keeping the stuffed animal in the middle. Remind students to hold on tight and do not let the stuffed animal fall off due to releasing the loop.

Goodbye

Sit in front of the students and greet each child individually. Provide augmentative communication or choice board for students that need assistance responding. Encourage eye contact as appropriate. Fleeting eye contact is acceptable is the intent is to provide joint attention.

Direct Instruction Example
Teacher/Therapist: "It's time for us to end group time. "Goodbye Mrs. X!"
Teacher/Therapist: "Goodbye Mrs. X!" (or Hi puppet name)

Verbal Response
Teacher/Therapist: "It's time for us to end group time. Goodbye student x!"
Student X: "Goodbye Mrs. X. (or Hi puppet name)

Non Verbal Response
Teacher/Therapist: "It's time for us to end group time. Goodbye student x!"
Student X: Initiate eye contact, wave, smile in direction of teacher/therapist/puppet

Use of Communication Device
Teacher/Therapist: "It's time for us to end group time. Goodbye student x!"
Student X: Touch "Goodbye Mrs. X" on given choice board, communication device, Ipad, etc.

Focus:
Gross motor skills
Follow directions
Extension arms

Materials:
Tug of War Rope

Method:

Greeting

Sit in front of the students and greet each child individually. Provide augmentative communication or choice board for students that need assistance responding. Encourage eye contact as appropriate. Fleeting eye contact is acceptable is the intent is to provide joint attention.

Direct Instruction Example
Teacher/Therapist: "It's time for us to have group time. Hi Mrs. X!"
Teacher/Therapist: "Hi Mrs. X!" (or Hi puppet name)

Verbal Response
Teacher/Therapist: "It's time for us to have group time. Hi student x!"
Student X: "Hi Mrs. X. (or Hi puppet name)

Non Verbal Response
Teacher/Therapist: "It's time for us to have group time. Hi student x!"
Student X: Initiate eye contact, wave, smile in direction of teacher/therapist/puppet

Use of Communication Device
Teacher/Therapist: "It's time for us to have group time. Hi student x!"
Student X: Touch "Hi Mrs. X" on given choice board, communication device, Ipad, etc.

Activity: Tug of War
Demonstrate holding on the rope with both hands using a supinated suitcase grasp and pull against each other on opposing sides.

Goodbye

Sit in front of the students and greet each child individually. Provide augmentative communication or choice board for students that need assistance responding. Encourage eye contact as appropriate. Fleeting eye contact is acceptable is the intent is to provide joint attention.

Direct Instruction Example
Teacher/Therapist: "It's time for us to end group time. "Goodbye Mrs. X!"
Teacher/Therapist: "Goodbye Mrs. X!" (or Hi puppet name)

Verbal Response
Teacher/Therapist: "It's time for us to end group time. Goodbye student x!"
Student X: "Goodbye Mrs. X. (or Hi puppet name)

Non Verbal Response
Teacher/Therapist: "It's time for us to end group time. Goodbye student x!"
Student X: Initiate eye contact, wave, smile in direction of teacher/therapist/puppet

Use of Communication Device
Teacher/Therapist: "It's time for us to end group time. Goodbye student x!"
Student X: Touch "Goodbye Mrs. X" on given choice board, communication device, Ipad, etc.

Focus:
In hand manipulation
Fine motor control
Eye hand coordination
Muscle gradation

Materials:
Bag of oranges cut into halves
Bowl
Paper Cups

Method:

Greeting

Sit in front of the students and greet each child individually. Provide augmentative communication or choice board for students that need assistance responding. Encourage eye contact as appropriate. Fleeting eye contact is acceptable is the intent is to provide joint attention.

Direct Instruction Example
Teacher/Therapist: "It's time for us to have group time. Hi Mrs. X!"
Teacher/Therapist: "Hi Mrs. X!" (or Hi puppet name)

Verbal Response
Teacher/Therapist: "It's time for us to have group time. Hi student x!"
Student X: "Hi Mrs. X. (or Hi puppet name)

Non Verbal Response
Teacher/Therapist: "It's time for us to have group time. Hi student x!"
Student X: Initiate eye contact, wave, smile in direction of teacher/therapist/puppet

Use of Communication Device
Teacher/Therapist: "It's time for us to have group time. Hi student x!"
Student X: Touch "Hi Mrs. X" on given choice board, communication device, Ipad, etc.

Demonstrate how to squeeze the orange and watch the juice release from the orange into the bowl.

Provide each student his own orange half to squeeze into the bowl.

After all are squeeze, pour a small amount of juice into paper cups to taste.

Goodbye

Sit in front of the students and greet each child individually. Provide augmentative communication or choice board for students that need assistance responding. Encourage eye contact as appropriate. Fleeting eye contact is acceptable is the intent is to provide joint attention.

Direct Instruction Example

Teacher/Therapist: "It's time for us to end group time. "Goodbye Mrs. X!"

Teacher/Therapist: "Goodbye Mrs. X!" (or Hi puppet name)

Verbal Response

Teacher/Therapist: "It's time for us to end group time. Goodbye student x!"

Student X: "Goodbye Mrs. X. (or Hi puppet name)

Non Verbal Response

Teacher/Therapist: "It's time for us to end group time. Goodbye student x!"

Student X: Initiate eye contact, wave, smile in direction of teacher/therapist/puppet

Use of Communication Device

Teacher/Therapist: "It's time for us to end group time. Goodbye student x!"

Student X: Touch "Goodbye Mrs. X" on given choice board, communication device, Ipad, etc.

Focus:
Tactile identification
Tactile discrimination
Fine motor manipulation

Materials:
Container with beans or sand
Small items (cars, plastic figures, etc. that are of child's interest)

Method:

Greeting

Sit in front of the students and greet each child individually. Provide augmentative communication or choice board for students that need assistance responding. Encourage eye contact as appropriate. Fleeting eye contact is acceptable is the intent is to provide joint attention.

Direct Instruction Example
Teacher/Therapist: "It's time for us to have group time. Hi Mrs. X!"
Teacher/Therapist: "Hi Mrs. X!" (or Hi puppet name)

Verbal Response
Teacher/Therapist: "It's time for us to have group time. Hi student x!"
Student X: "Hi Mrs. X. (or Hi puppet name)

Non Verbal Response
Teacher/Therapist: "It's time for us to have group time. Hi student x!"
Student X: Initiate eye contact, wave, smile in direction of teacher/therapist/puppet

Use of Communication Device
Teacher/Therapist: "It's time for us to have group time. Hi student x!"
Student X: Touch "Hi Mrs. X" on given choice board, communication device, Ipad, etc.

Hide items in the sand/bean box. Have student search for items in the box and manipulate the sand/beans to obtain objects.

Goodbye

Sit in front of the students and greet each child individually. Provide augmentative communication or choice board for students that need assistance responding. Encourage eye contact as appropriate. Fleeting eye contact is acceptable is the intent is to provide joint attention.

Direct Instruction Example
Teacher/Therapist: "It's time for us to end group time. "Goodbye Mrs. X!"
Teacher/Therapist: "Goodbye Mrs. X!" (or Hi puppet name)

Verbal Response
Teacher/Therapist: "It's time for us to end group time. Goodbye student x!"
Student X: "Goodbye Mrs. X. (or Hi puppet name)

Non Verbal Response
Teacher/Therapist: "It's time for us to end group time. Goodbye student x!"
Student X: Initiate eye contact, wave, smile in direction of teacher/therapist/puppet

Use of Communication Device
Teacher/Therapist: "It's time for us to end group time. Goodbye student x!"
Student X: Touch "Goodbye Mrs. X" on given choice board, communication device, Ipad, etc.

Focus:
Motor planning
Shoulder girdle strength
Eye hand coordination
Muscle gradation and strengthening
Body Awareness

Materials:
Pillowcase
Beanbags
Obstacle Course

Method:

Greeting

Sit in front of the students and greet each child individually. Provide augmentative communication or choice board for students that need assistance responding. Encourage eye contact as appropriate. Fleeting eye contact is acceptable is the intent is to provide joint attention.

Direct Instruction Example
Teacher/Therapist: "It's time for us to have group time. Hi Mrs. X!"
Teacher/Therapist: "Hi Mrs. X!" (or Hi puppet name)

Verbal Response
Teacher/Therapist: "It's time for us to have group time. Hi student x!"
Student X: "Hi Mrs. X. (or Hi puppet name)

Non Verbal Response
Teacher/Therapist: "It's time for us to have group time. Hi student x!"
Student X: Initiate eye contact, wave, smile in direction of teacher/therapist/puppet

Use of Communication Device
Teacher/Therapist: "It's time for us to have group time. Hi student x!"
Student X: Touch "Hi Mrs. X" on given choice board, communication device, Ipad, etc.

Prior to play, put beanbags in pillow case and secure it closed (sew or tied).

Demonstrate a four point stance. Have a teacher assist and place the pillow on your back. While in four point and with the pillow on the back, demonstrate crawling like a turtle.

While the child is in the four point, place the pillow case on his back.

Have the student first crawl back and forth in a cleared area. Then to expand the play, have the student crawl through a obstacle course while trying to keep the pillow case on the back.

Goodbye

Sit in front of the students and greet each child individually. Provide augmentative communication or choice board for students that need assistance responding. Encourage eye contact as appropriate. Fleeting eye contact is acceptable is the intent is to provide joint attention.

Direct Instruction Example
Teacher/Therapist: "It's time for us to end group time. "Goodbye Mrs. X!"
Teacher/Therapist: "Goodbye Mrs. X!" (or Hi puppet name)

Verbal Response
Teacher/Therapist: "It's time for us to end group time. Goodbye student x!"
Student X: "Goodbye Mrs. X. (or Hi puppet name)

Non Verbal Response
Teacher/Therapist: "It's time for us to end group time. Goodbye student x!"
Student X: Initiate eye contact, wave, smile in direction of teacher/therapist/puppet

Use of Communication Device
Teacher/Therapist: "It's time for us to end group time. Goodbye student x!"
Student X: Touch "Goodbye Mrs. X" on given choice board, communication device, Ipad, etc.

Focus:
Muscle control
Follow direction
Proprioception

Materials:
Green and red construction paper

Method:

Greeting

Sit in front of the students and greet each child individually. Provide augmentative communication or choice board for students that need assistance responding. Encourage eye contact as appropriate. Fleeting eye contact is acceptable is the intent is to provide joint attention.

Direct Instruction Example
Teacher/Therapist: "It's time for us to have group time. Hi Mrs. X!"
Teacher/Therapist: "Hi Mrs. X!" (or Hi puppet name)

Verbal Response
Teacher/Therapist: "It's time for us to have group time. Hi student x!"
Student X: "Hi Mrs. X. (or Hi puppet name)

Non Verbal Response
Teacher/Therapist: "It's time for us to have group time. Hi student x!"
Student X: Initiate eye contact, wave, smile in direction of teacher/therapist/puppet

Use of Communication Device
Teacher/Therapist: "It's time for us to have group time. Hi student x!"
Student X: Touch "Hi Mrs. X" on given choice board, communication device, Ipad, etc.

Activity: Stop and Go
Teach red and green as representing "stop" and "go".

If student is unable to understanding representational pictures, simply use verbal instruction.

If student is unable to understand differences between verbal instructions "stop" and "go", adapt this activity to teach stop and go using physical instruction for the concepts.
To teach go: Hold child's hand when running, walking fast or wheeling. Constantly reinforce "go" by saying "green means go" or simply "go".

To teach stop: Over exaggerate stopping and say "stop" or "red means stop"

Once child understand go/stop or green/red meaning go/stop, you can play a race game. Have a teacher hold colored paper and call out the appropriate command "stop" or "go". Students will move or stop depending on the direction.

Goodbye

Sit in front of the students and greet each child individually. Provide augmentative communication or choice board for students that need assistance responding. Encourage eye contact as appropriate. Fleeting eye contact is acceptable is the intent is to provide joint attention.

Direct Instruction Example
Teacher/Therapist: "It's time for us to end group time. "Goodbye Mrs. X!"
Teacher/Therapist: "Goodbye Mrs. X!" (or Hi puppet name)

Verbal Response
Teacher/Therapist: "It's time for us to end group time. Goodbye student x!"
Student X: "Goodbye Mrs. X. (or Hi puppet name)

Non Verbal Response
Teacher/Therapist: "It's time for us to end group time. Goodbye student x!"
Student X: Initiate eye contact, wave, smile in direction of teacher/therapist/puppet

Use of Communication Device
Teacher/Therapist: "It's time for us to end group time. Goodbye student x!"
Student X: Touch "Goodbye Mrs. X" on given choice board, communication device, Ipad, etc.

Week 24

Focus:
Balance
Joint Attention

Materials:
Tactile ball (koosh, sensory, hacky sack)

Method:

Greeting

Sit in front of the students and greet each child individually. Provide augmentative communication or choice board for students that need assistance responding. Encourage eye contact as appropriate. Fleeting eye contact is acceptable is the intent is to provide joint attention.

Direct Instruction Example
Teacher/Therapist: "It's time for us to have group time. Hi Mrs. X!"
Teacher/Therapist: "Hi Mrs. X!" (or Hi puppet name)

Verbal Response
Teacher/Therapist: "It's time for us to have group time. Hi student x!"
Student X: "Hi Mrs. X. (or Hi puppet name)

Non Verbal Response
Teacher/Therapist: "It's time for us to have group time. Hi student x!"
Student X: Initiate eye contact, wave, smile in direction of teacher/therapist/puppet

Use of Communication Device
Teacher/Therapist: "It's time for us to have group time. Hi student x!"
Student X: Touch "Hi Mrs. X" on given choice board, communication device, Ipad, etc.

Activity: Ball Balancing

Place and balance the ball on the head.

While the ball is on the head, make faces to the child and have them attempt to reproduce the faces.

Keep the ball steady despite moving facial parts.

Goodbye

Sit in front of the students and greet each child individually. Provide augmentative communication or choice board for students that need assistance responding. Encourage eye contact as appropriate. Fleeting eye contact is acceptable is the intent is to provide joint attention.

Direct Instruction Example
Teacher/Therapist: "It's time for us to end group time. "Goodbye Mrs. X!"
Teacher/Therapist: "Goodbye Mrs. X!" (or Hi puppet name)

Verbal Response
Teacher/Therapist: "It's time for us to end group time. Goodbye student x!"
Student X: "Goodbye Mrs. X. (or Hi puppet name)

Non Verbal Response
Teacher/Therapist: "It's time for us to end group time. Goodbye student x!"
Student X: Initiate eye contact, wave, smile in direction of teacher/therapist/puppet

Use of Communication Device
Teacher/Therapist: "It's time for us to end group time. Goodbye student x!"
Student X: Touch "Goodbye Mrs. X" on given choice board, communication device, Ipad, etc.

Focus:
Balance
Gross Motor
Muscle Control

Materials:
Six beanbags
Bucket

Method:

Greeting

Sit in front of the students and greet each child individually. Provide augmentative communication or choice board for students that need assistance responding. Encourage eye contact as appropriate. Fleeting eye contact is acceptable is the intent is to provide joint attention.

Direct Instruction Example
Teacher/Therapist: "It's time for us to have group time. Hi Mrs. X!"
Teacher/Therapist: "Hi Mrs. X!" (or Hi puppet name)

Verbal Response
Teacher/Therapist: "It's time for us to have group time. Hi student x!"
Student X: "Hi Mrs. X. (or Hi puppet name)

Non Verbal Response
Teacher/Therapist: "It's time for us to have group time. Hi student x!"
Student X: Initiate eye contact, wave, smile in direction of teacher/therapist/puppet

Use of Communication Device
Teacher/Therapist: "It's time for us to have group time. Hi student x!"
Student X: Touch "Hi Mrs. X" on given choice board, communication device, Ipad, etc.

Activity: Beanbag Toss on Bucket

Have the child walk in a straight line toward the bucket.

Once the child is about 1 feet away from bucket, cue them to toss the bean bag in the bucket. Continue practicing as the distance between the bucket and toss location is increased.

Goodbye

Sit in front of the students and greet each child individually. Provide augmentative communication or choice board for students that need assistance responding. Encourage eye contact as appropriate. Fleeting eye contact is acceptable is the intent is to provide joint attention.

Direct Instruction Example
Teacher/Therapist: "It's time for us to end group time. "Goodbye Mrs. X!"
Teacher/Therapist: "Goodbye Mrs. X!" (or Hi puppet name)

Verbal Response
Teacher/Therapist: "It's time for us to end group time. Goodbye student x!"
Student X: "Goodbye Mrs. X. (or Hi puppet name)

Non Verbal Response
Teacher/Therapist: "It's time for us to end group time. Goodbye student x!"
Student X: Initiate eye contact, wave, smile in direction of teacher/therapist/puppet

Use of Communication Device
Teacher/Therapist: "It's time for us to end group time. Goodbye student x!"
Student X: Touch "Goodbye Mrs. X" on given choice board, communication device, Ipad, etc.

References

American Occupational Therapy Association. (2008). Occupational therapy practice framework: Domain and process (2nd ed.). American Journal of Occupational Therapy , 62, 625–683.

American Occupational Therapy Association (2012). Role of Occupational Therapy with Children and Youth with Children and Youth in School in School-Based Practice.

Ayres, A. J. (2005). *Sensory integration and the child: 25th anniversary edition.* Lost Angeles, CA: Western Psychological Services.

Individuals With Disabilities Education Act, 20 U.S.C. § 1400 (2004).

National Governors Association Center for Best Practices & Council of Chief State School Officers. (2010). *Common Core State Standards.* Washington, DC: Authors.

Please check out our other Purple Toes Books for your Occupational Therapy needs.

Http://www.purpletoesbooks.com

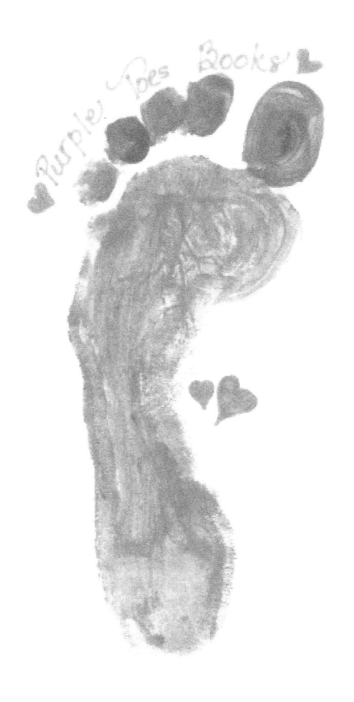

Purple Toes Books

Made in the USA
Monee, IL
12 October 2022

15746120R00057